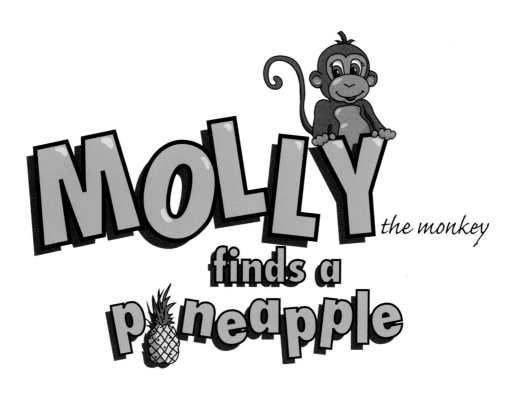

# MOLLY *the monkey*
## finds a p neapple

By Kathleen Stefancin, M.S., R.D.
Illustrated by Patricia Popovich, M.A., A.T.

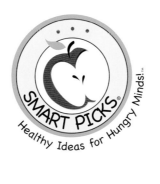

SMART PICKS®
Healthy Ideas for Hungry Minds!™

## Dedication

To my family and the next generation, stay connected to the healing power of plants by eating fruits and vegetables! ~ K.S.

To my parents, thank you for introducing me to the magic and wonder of the natural world! - and Kathleen, thank you for believing in me - you are an amazing woman!  ~ P.P.

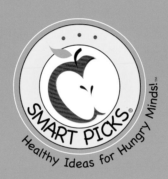

Smart Picks, Inc., P.O. Box 771440 Lakewood, Ohio 44107
or visit:
www.smartpicks.com

ISBN 978-0-9764785-4-6

Library of Congress Control Number: 2009907332
Copyright © 2010 by Kathleen Stefancin
All Rights Reserved. Self-published by Kathleen Stefancin.

Printed by Blue Ocean Printing, Anaheim, California, USA

Printed in China
Book design, cover art and all illustrations by Patricia Popovich

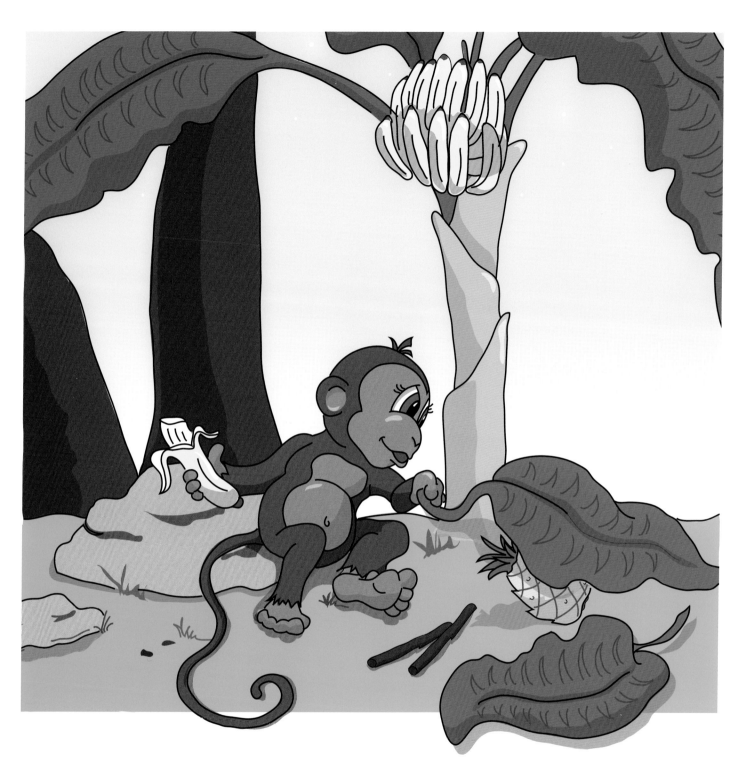

**While sitting under her favorite banana plant one summer day, Molly the monkey suddenly noticed a pineapple lying under a large green leaf.**

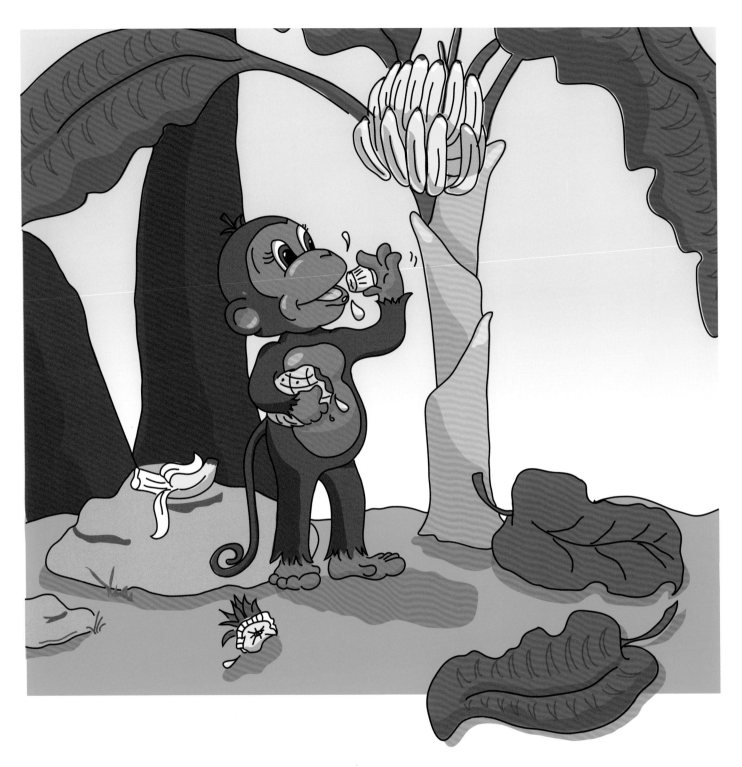

Curious, Molly picked up the pineapple and tried a piece.
"Delicious!" she shouted. Then she ate the rest of
the sweet, juicy pineapple.

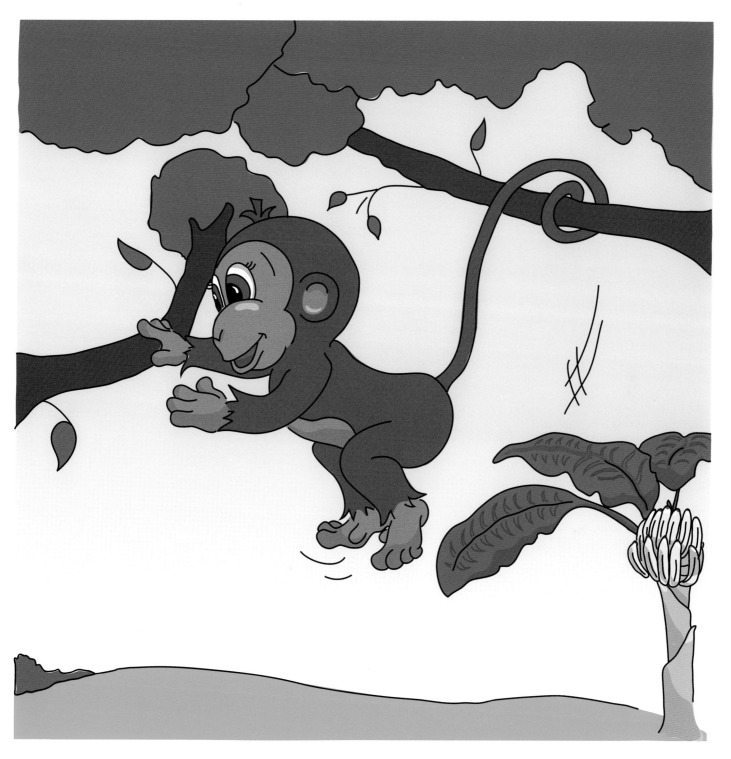

Believing the pineapple had fallen from a tree,
Molly began to swing from branch to branch,
looking for more pineapples to eat.

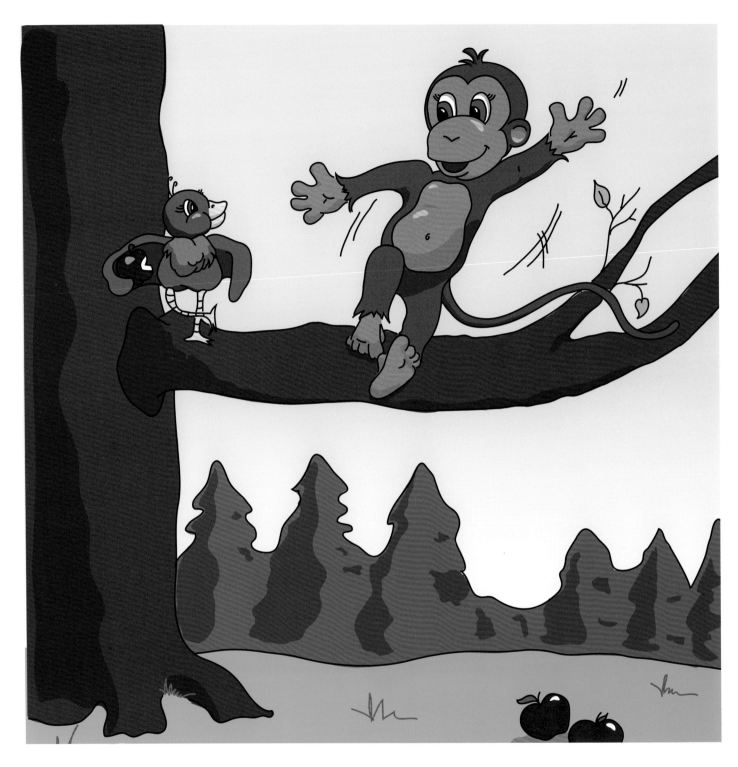

**Along the way she met a pretty little bluebird snacking on an apple. "Good morning, Miss Bluebird", said Molly. "Do pineapples grow on trees?"**

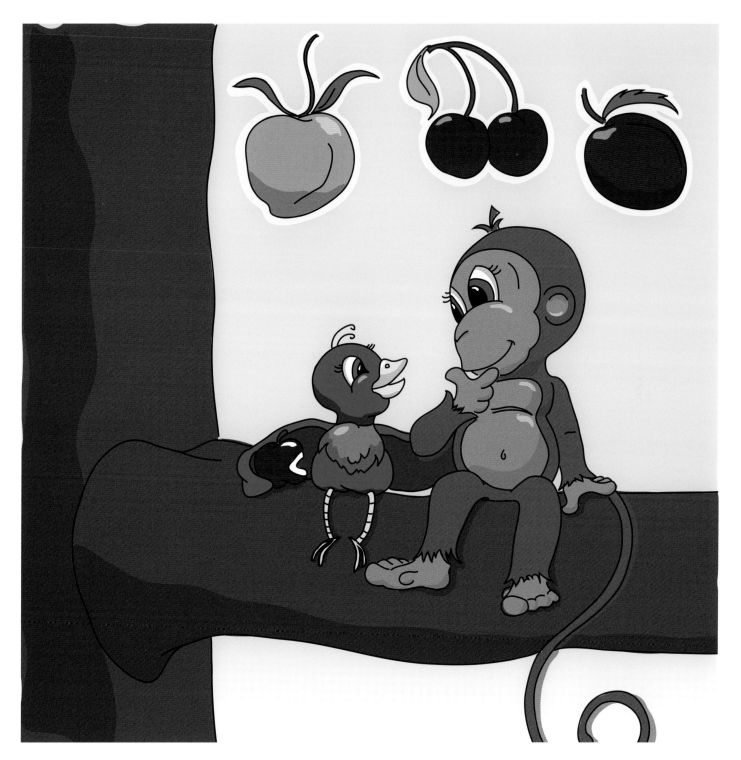

Miss Bluebird replied, "Oh no, pineapples don't grow on trees, like peaches, cherries and plums! I think pineapples grow on vines."

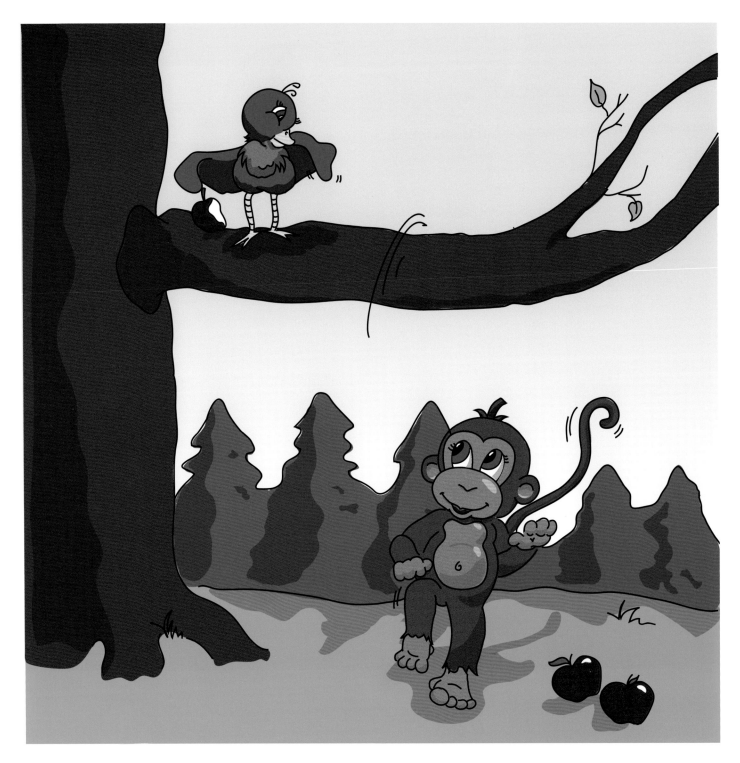

Molly thanked Miss Bluebird and jumped to the ground.
She skipped through the forest, hoping to find a
pineapple growing on a vine.

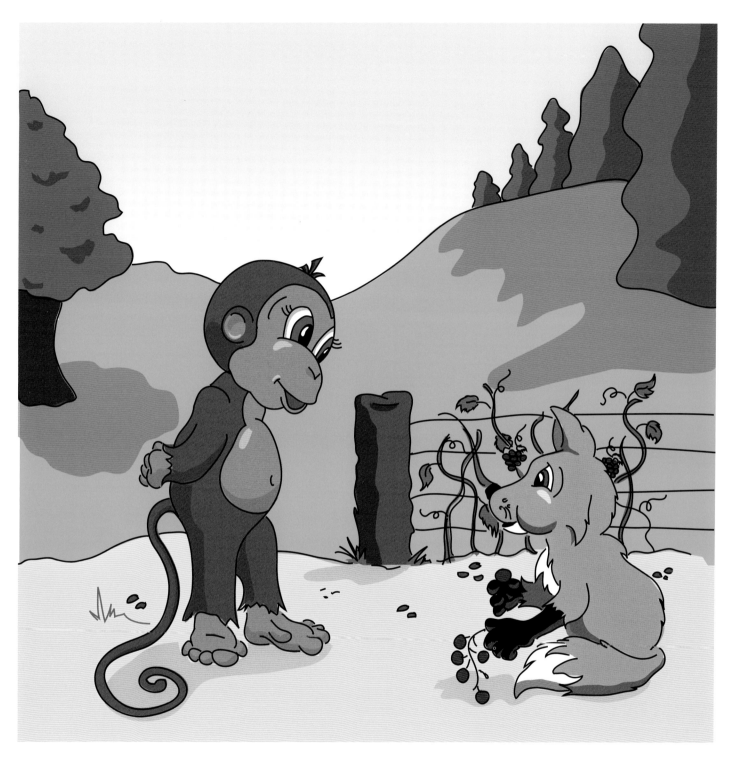

As she approached a small patch of vines, she saw a
red fox nibbling on some grapes. "Hello, Mr. Fox," said Molly.
"Do pineapples grow on vines?"

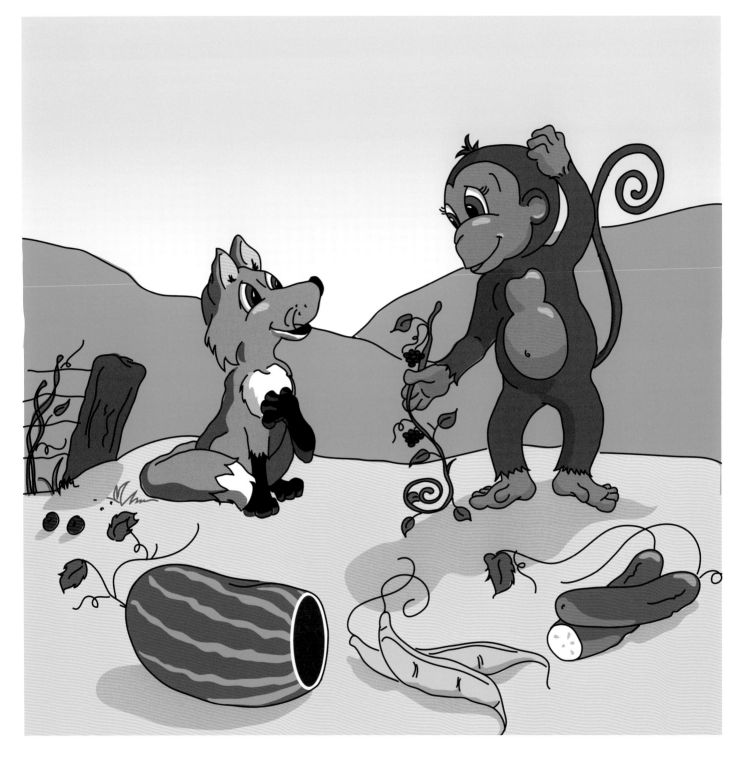

Mr. Fox replied, "Oh no. Pineapples don't grow on vines like watermelons, green beans and cucumbers!
I believe pineapples grow on bushes."

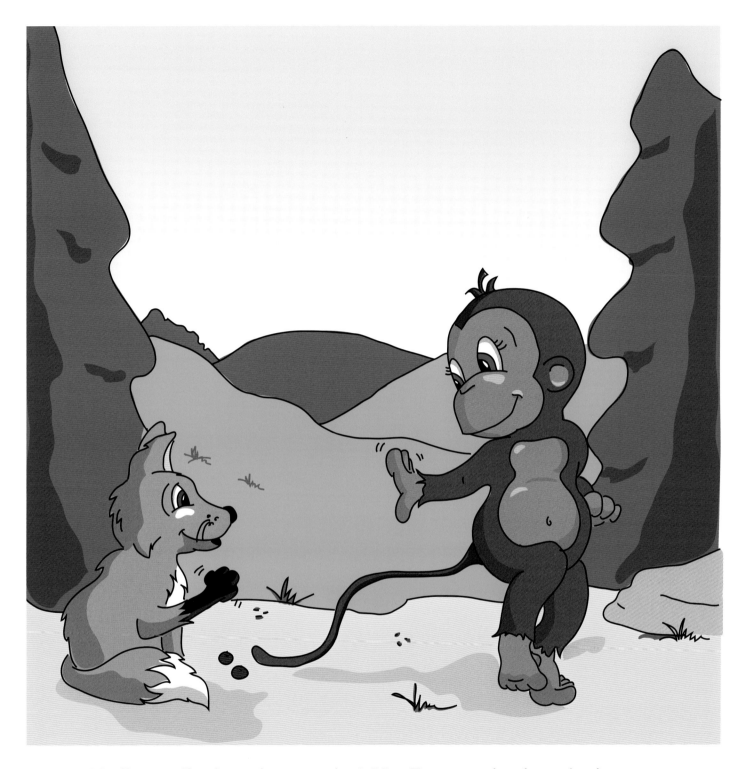

**Molly smiled and waved at Mr. Fox as she hurried away in search of a pineapple. She was determined to find one.**

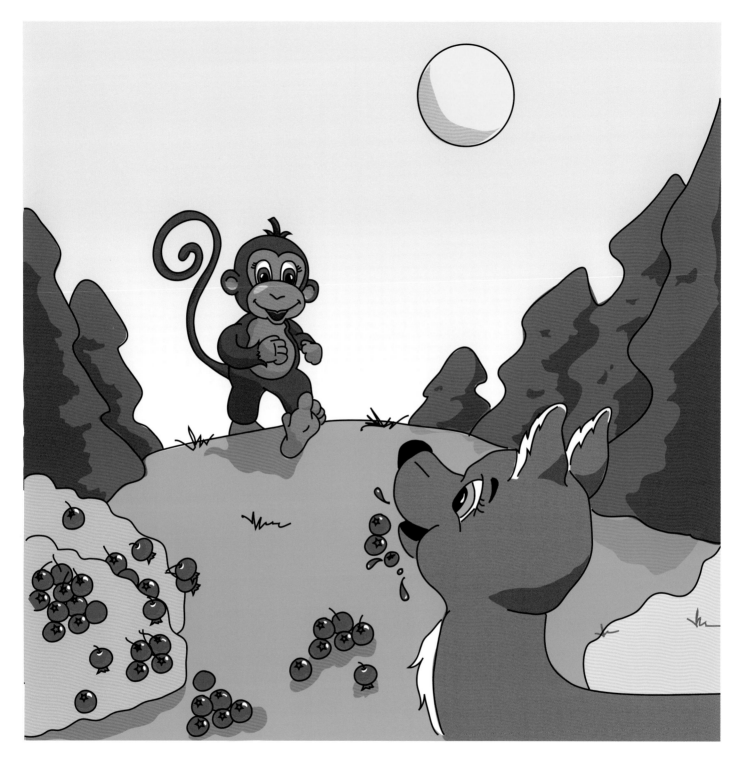

Across a small field, Molly saw a cluster of brightly colored bushes. As she reached the bushes, she noticed a beautiful deer, chewing a mouthful of blueberries. "Good afternoon, Miss Deer," said Molly. "Are there any pineapples growing on these bushes?"

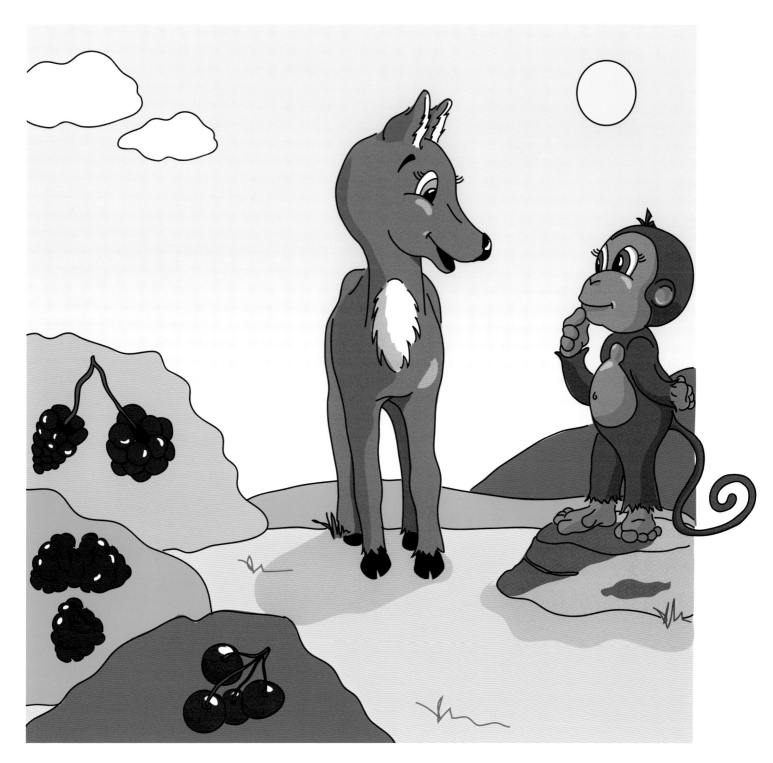

Miss Deer replied, "Oh no. Pineapples don't grow on bushes like blackberries, red raspberries, and cranberries! I bet pineapples grow in the ground."

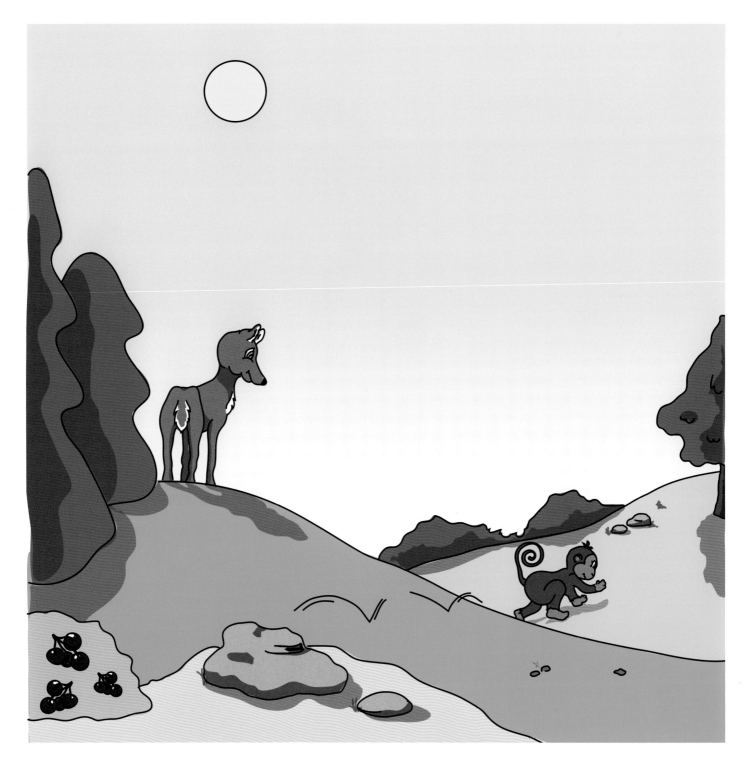

Molly said good-bye to Miss Deer and trotted away.
She stared at the ground so she didn't miss a
single trace of pineapple.

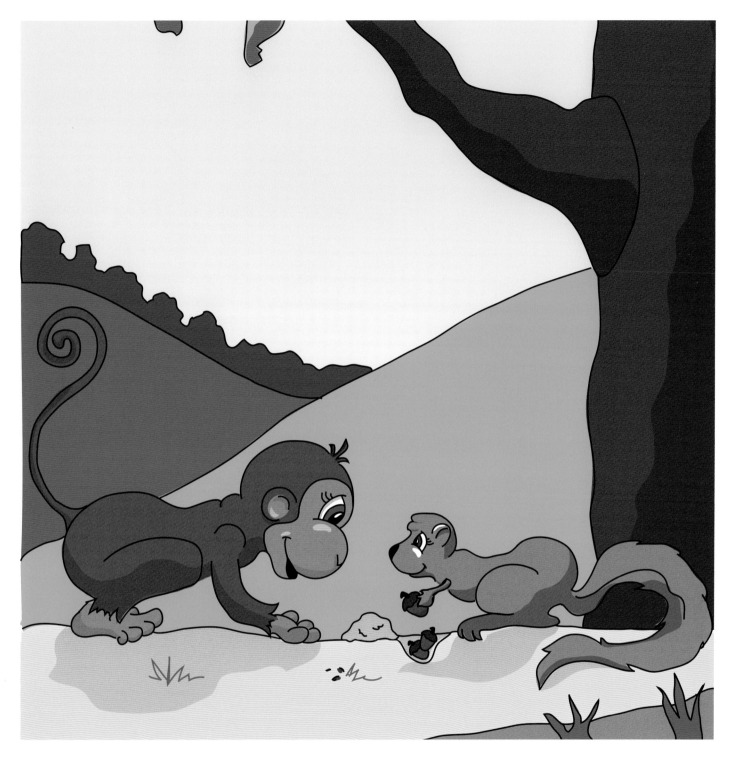

Eventually, she came face to face with a red squirrel busily hiding nuts in the ground. "Hi, Miss Squirrel," said Molly. "Have you seen any pineapples growing in the ground?"

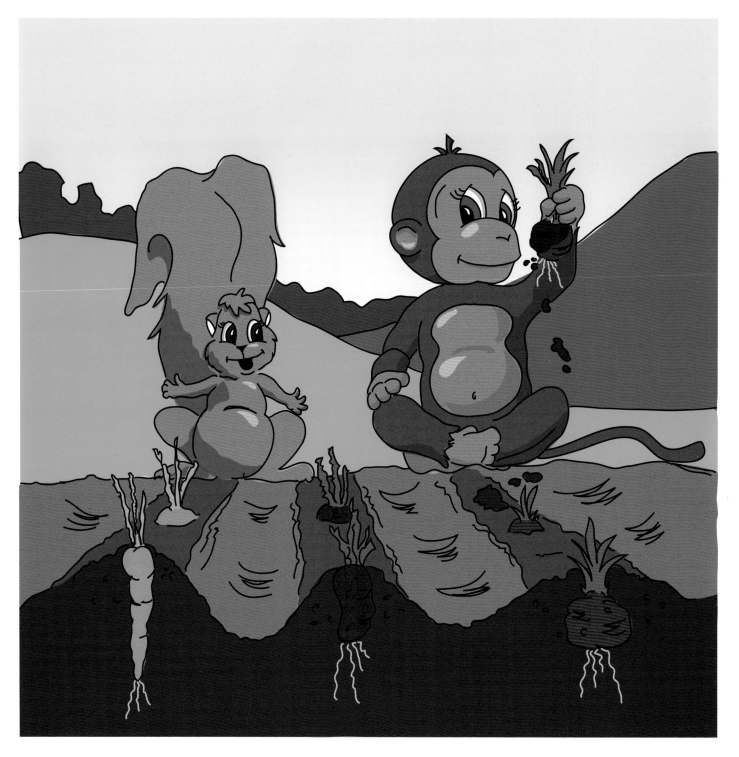

Miss Squirrel replied, "Oh no. Pineapples don't grow
in the ground like carrots, sweet potatoes, and beets!
I imagine pineapples grow on top of the ground."

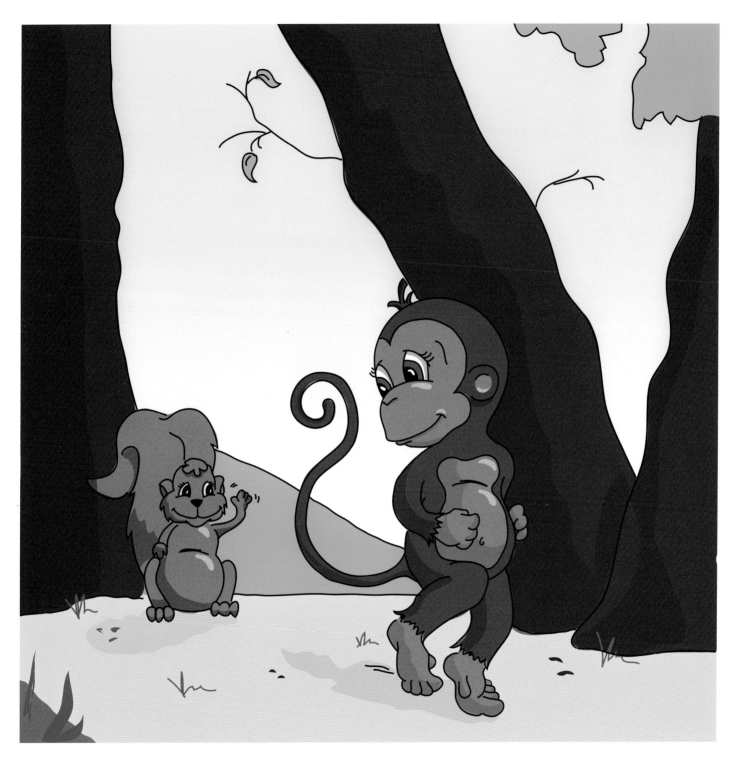

Molly wanted a pineapple more than ever.
She nodded a thank-you to Miss Squirrel and hurried by her.
Molly knew she was getting closer to discovering
where pineapples grew.

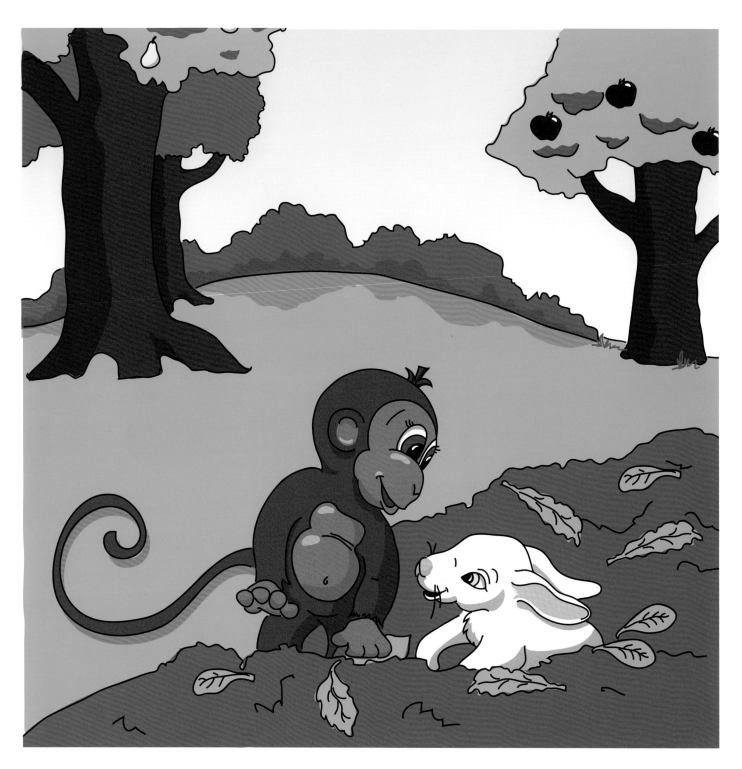

Next, she came across a valley of leafy greens. As she walked
through the greens, a rabbit hopped up to her and said,
" Hello my friend are you looking for something?" "Hi, Mr. Rabbit,"
said Molly. "I'm looking for a pineapple. Have you seen one
growing on top of the ground among these leafy greens?"

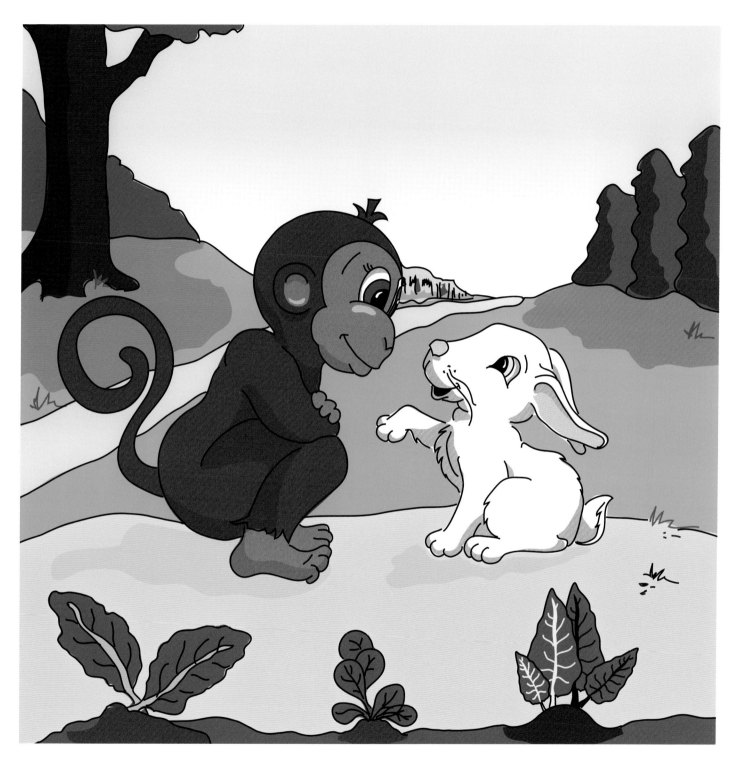

Mr. Rabbit replied, "Oh no. Pineapples don't grow on top of the ground like kale, spinach and Swiss chard! I picture pineapples growing on a stalk."

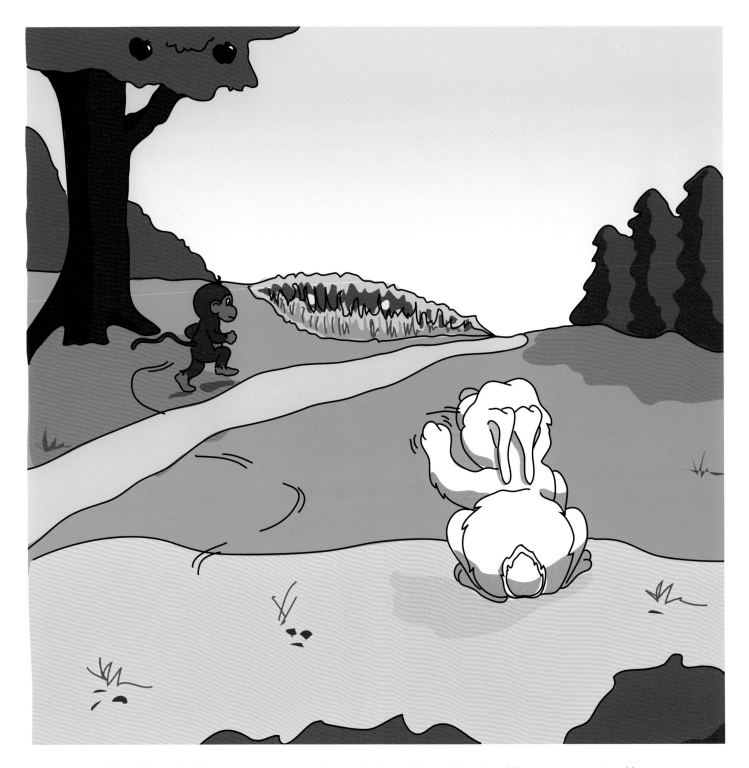

Mr. Rabbit turned and pointed to the tall green stalks across the river. Excited, Molly leaped to the other side of the river. She ran towards the stalks, thinking she'd finally found a pineapple.

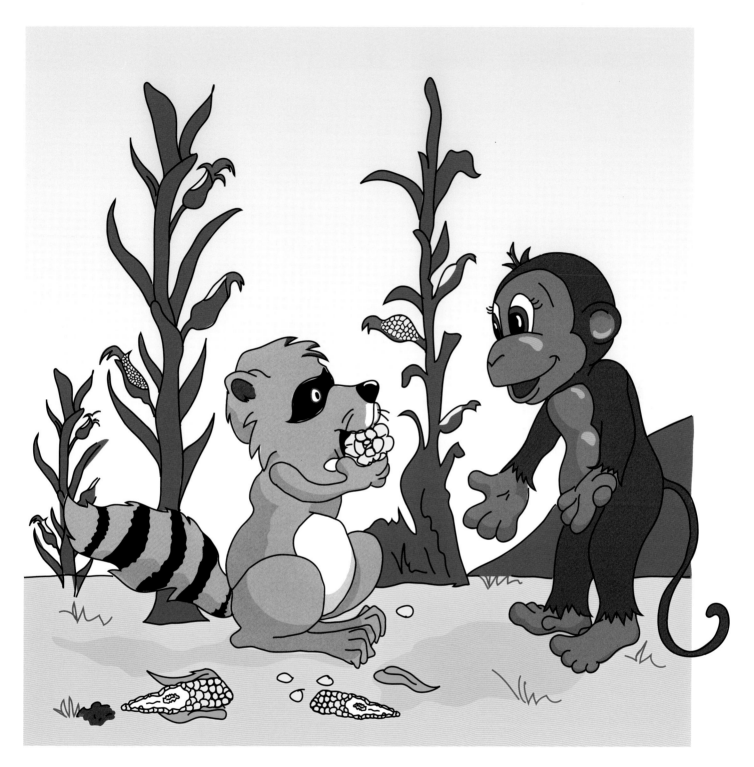

When she reached the stalks, she spotted a big raccoon eating yellow corn. "Mr. Raccoon," she said, out of breath, "where are the pineapples?"

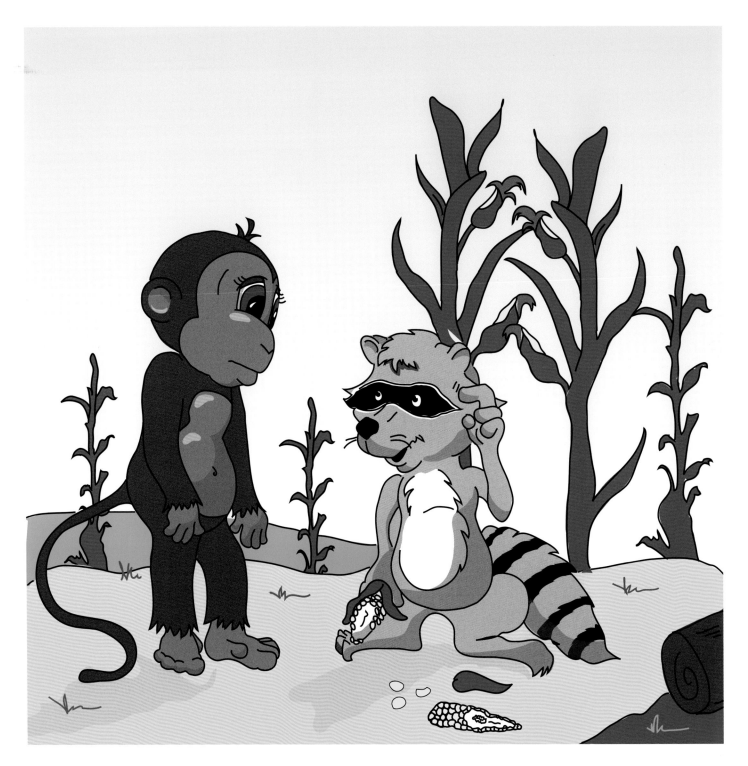

Mr. Raccoon replied, "Oh no. Pineapples don't grow on stalks like corn." He scratched his head. "In fact, I'm not sure where pineapples grow." Molly felt very disappointed.

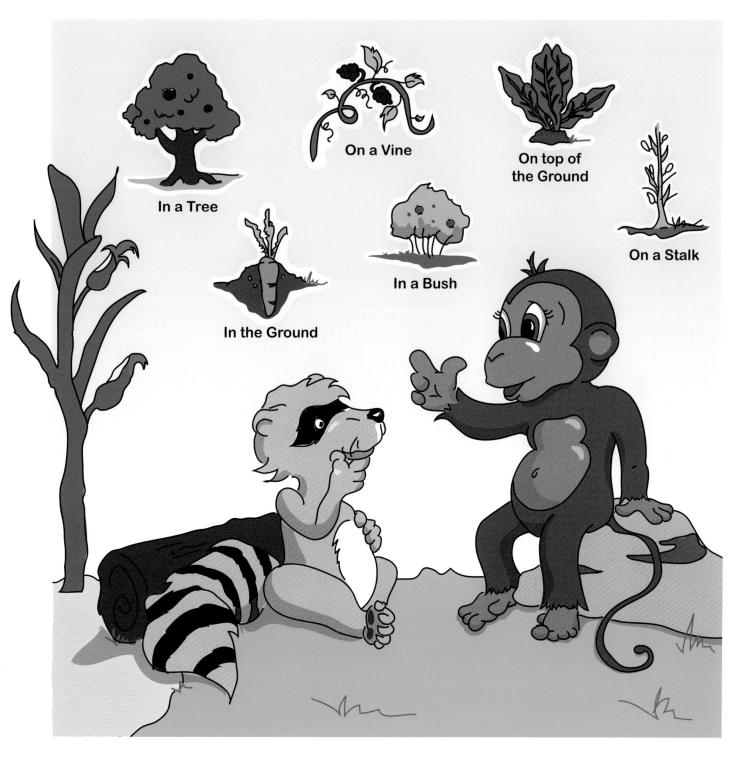

She explained to Mr. Raccoon, "I've looked for a pineapple in a tree, on a vine, and in a bush. I've searched in the ground, on top of the ground, and on a stalk."

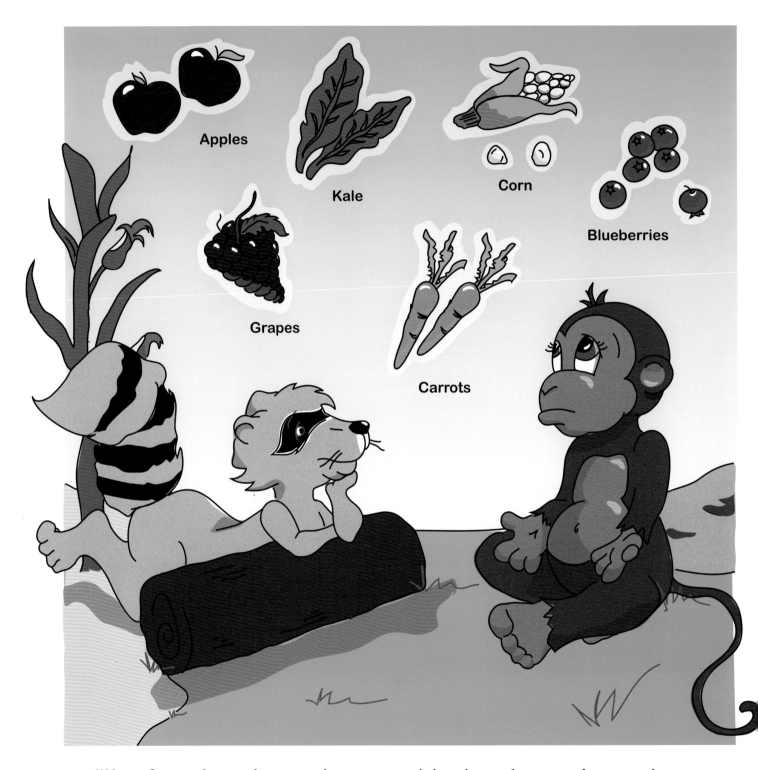

"I've found apples and grapes, blueberries and carrots, and kale and corn. But I still haven't found a pineapple." She sighed. Molly thanked Mr. Raccoon and wondered what to do next.

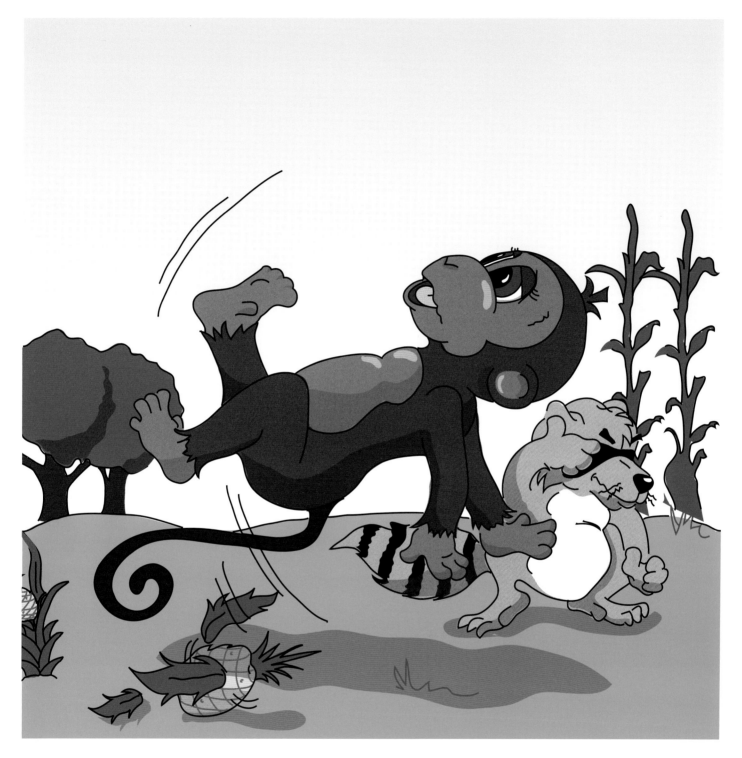

As she turned to leave, she slipped on something
round and hard, and landed on her back.

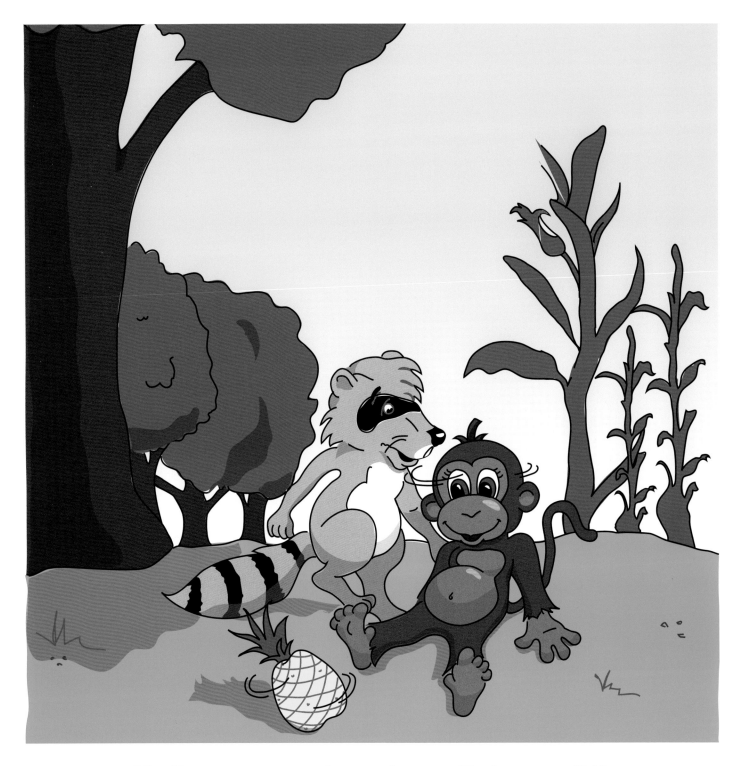

**Mr. Raccoon raced over to see if she was OK.
A little stunned, Molly sat up and a huge smile appeared on her
face. She'd finally found a pineapple!**

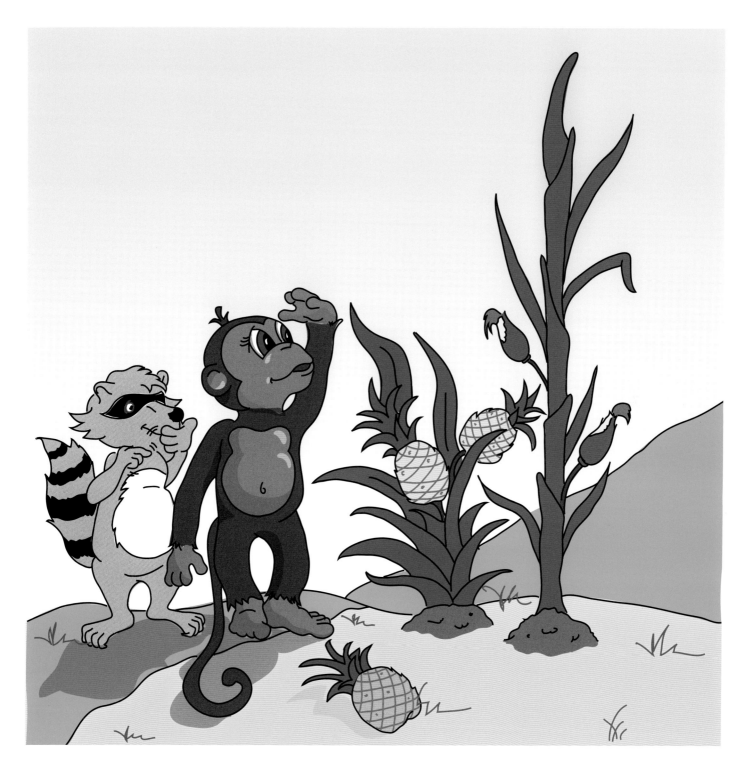

Molly was fascinated to discover that pineapples grew on plants that were only three feet high - no taller than her. Even Mr. Raccoon was surprised! Because he ate only corn, he didn't notice the pineapples growing next to the corn stalks.

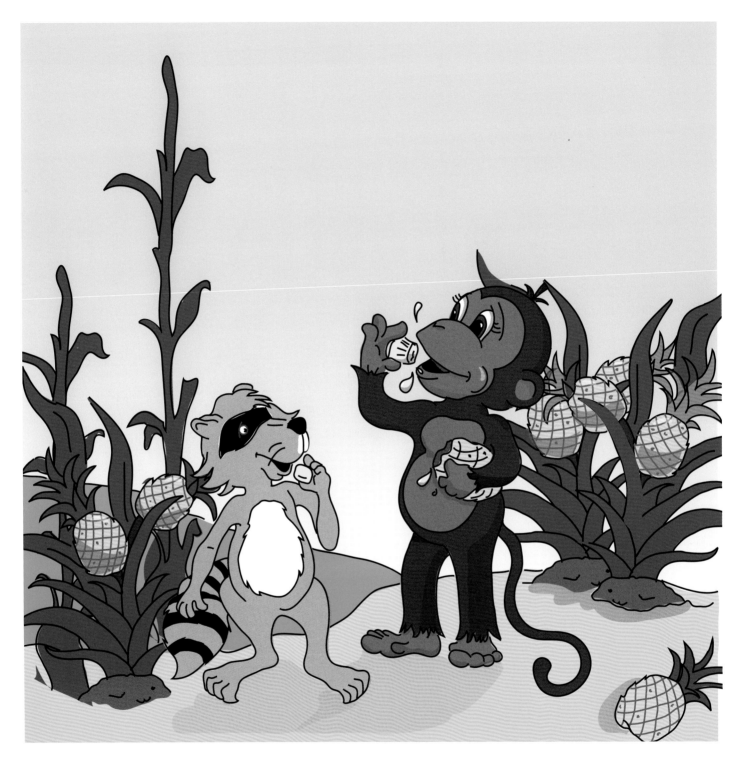

**Molly grabbed a fresh, juicy pineapple from the plant
and began to eat it. "Delicious!" she shouted, looking
around joyfully at all the pineapple plants.
Mr. Raccoon even tasted a bite.**

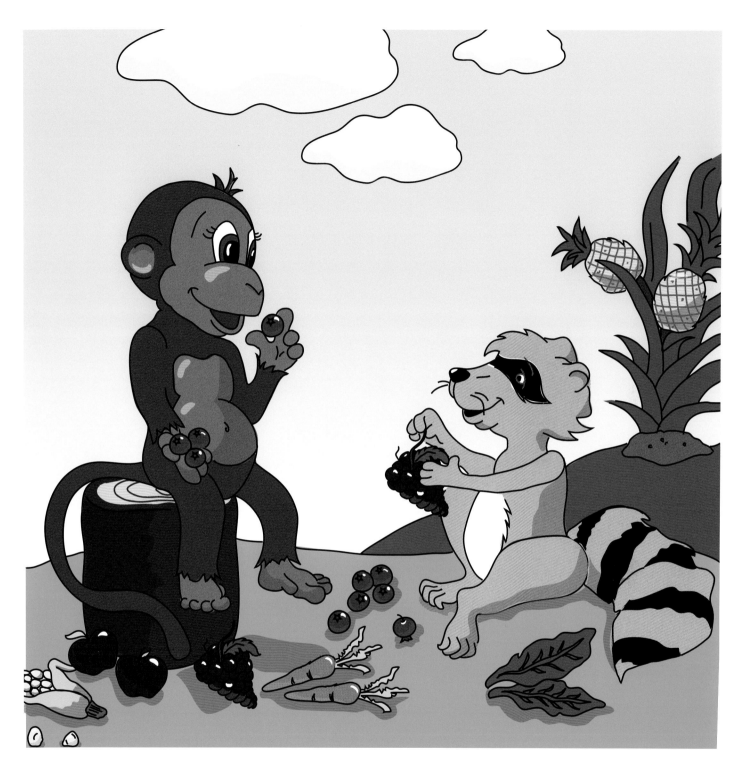

She thought about all the fruits and vegetables she'd found while looking for a pineapple. She decided to try some apples and grapes, blueberries and carrots, and kale and corn. Mr. Raccoon wanted to taste the other fruits and vegetables too.

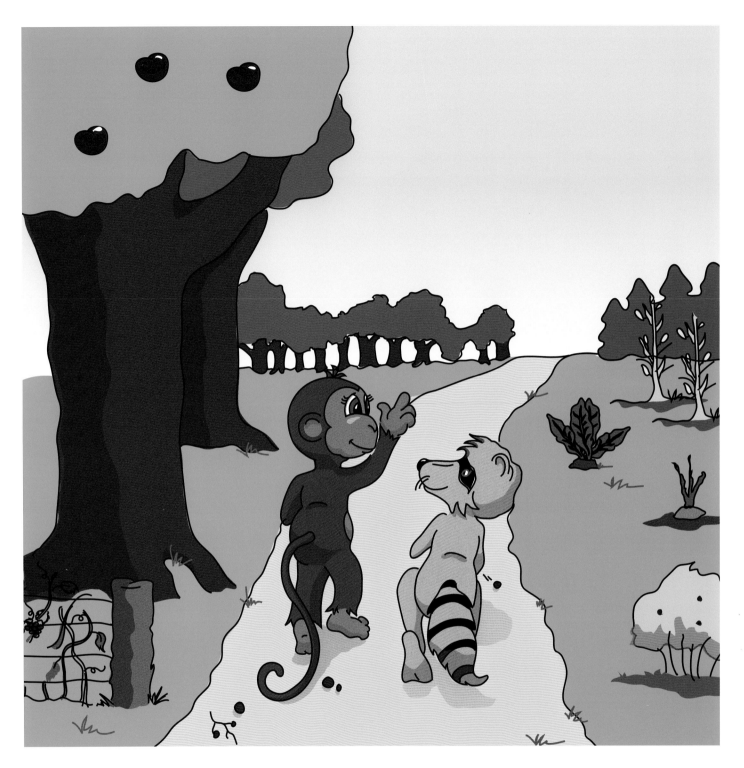

Molly and Mr. Raccoon became good friends,
and returned to all the places where Molly
had discovered the other fruits and vegetables.
They tasted every last one of them.

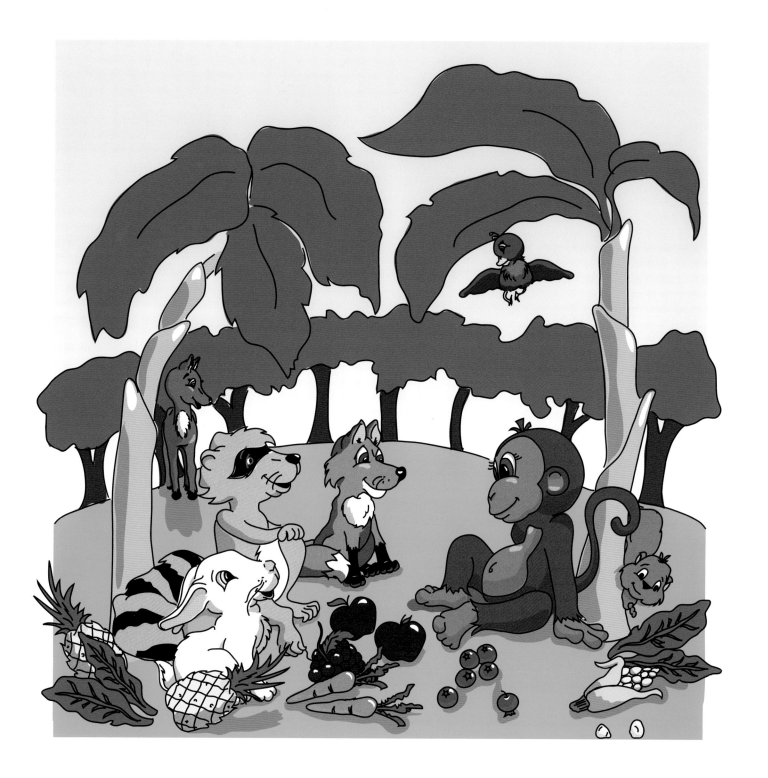

It wasn't long before all the animals in the forest were eating a variety of fruits and vegetables, thanks to Molly. Today, you'll often find Molly the monkey and her friends sitting under her favorite banana plant, surrounded by lots of fruits and vegetables.

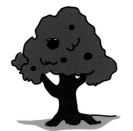

**In a Tree**

_____
_____
_____
_____
_____

_____
_____
_____
_____
_____

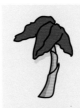

**On a Vine**

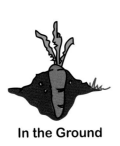

**On top of
the Ground**

_____
_____
_____
_____
_____

_____
_____
_____
_____
_____

**On a Bush**

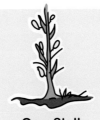

**In the Ground**

_____
_____
_____
_____
_____

_____
_____
_____
_____
_____

**On a Stalk**

# MOLLY
_the monkey_

## Molly's Activity Sheet

**Can you help Molly identify 5
more fruits and vegetables
for each category?**

**For a complete list of how
fruits & vegetables grow please visit:
www.smartpicks.com
and click on the
FREE Materials button.**

**All materials gathered from**
_Molly the Monkey Finds a Pineapple_

banana
pineapple
_____
_____
_____

**On a Plant**

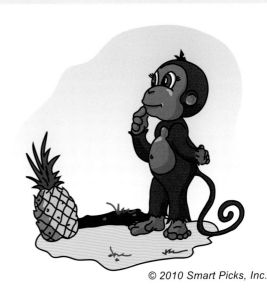